MOON PREP'S GUIDE TO MMI

FOR MEDICAL ADMISSIONS, DIRECT MEDICAL
PROGRAMS, BS/MD, AND BS/DO

KRISTEN MOON

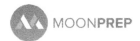

Copyright © 2022 by Kristen Moon, Moon Prep LLC

All rights reserved.

No part of this book may be reproduced in any form or by any electronic or mechanical means, including information storage and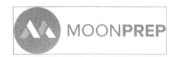
retrieval systems, without written permission from the author, except for the use of brief quotations in a book review.

Published by Moon Prep, ver. 1.2
www.moonprep.com

ISBN: 979-8-36-083873-9

ALSO BY KRISTEN MOON

BS/MD Programs: A Comprehensive Guide

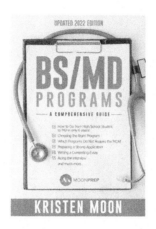

CONTENTS

Preface	vii
Author's Note	ix
1. INTRODUCTION TO THE MMI	1
2. HOW THIS BOOK WILL HELP YOU PREPARE	7
Common Misconceptions About the MMI	9
3. MMI STRATEGY DISCUSSION	13
Remember Your Communication Skills Are Always On Display	15
Other Strategic Choices You Can Make During Your MMI	16
How To Approach MMI Questions	19
Urgent Medical Treatment in Life-Threatening Situations	20
Medical Care Issues While Treating Minors	21
Ethical Guidance	22
4. SAMPLE MMI QUESTIONS FOR BS/MD AND MEDICAL SCHOOL STUDENTS, PART ONE	27
5. SAMPLE MMI QUESTIONS FOR MEDICAL SCHOOL STUDENTS, PART TWO	47
6. BE FULLY PREPARED FOR THE MMI	61
7. LIST OF MEDICAL SCHOOLS USING MMI IN THEIR ADMISSIONS PROCESS	65
About the Author	69
Also by Kristen Moon	71

PREFACE

In *Moon Prep's Guide to MMI: for Medical Admissions, Direct Medical Programs, BS/MD, and BS/DO*, you'll find detailed and up-to-date information on the critical MMI interview process. Feel confident about your Multiple Mini Interview (MMI); this guide covers all the critical details you need to know, including:

- MMI vs traditional interviews - understand the nuances
- What topics MMI is evaluating you on (and what it's not!)
- Virtual interviewing tips
- Specific tips for BS/MD students on how to prepare for the MMI
- What MMI questions are actually asking you
- How to ace the MMI interview
- Strategies for the different question types
- Which medical schools require the MMI

PREFACE

- Packed with 55+ sample questions, with analysis

AUTHOR'S NOTE

FEW CAREERS ARE AS CHALLENGING and rewarding as a life in medicine. For those ambitious students embarking on the road to medical school, all of us here at Moon Prep take great pride in our collective expertise and unique success rates in helping those dreams become a reality. From traditional paths to medicine to Direct Medical Programs, like the BS/MD and BS/DO alternatives, we partner with students and their families at every turn to ensure they successfully navigate the complex application requirements and the crucial interviews, such as the MMI (multiple mini-interview).

Every year, thousands of students compete for a limited amount of coveted seats at U.S. medical schools. The reality is that less than 50% of applicants will get accepted. Daunting, challenging, and nerve-racking are a few of the words we hear every year from our students. Moon Prep is dedicated to alleviating their concerns and streamlining the process with confidence, assembling a caring and trusted team of professionals that have helped countless students secure admission at some of the country's most competitive programs. These mentors and counselors—many current MD, DO, and joint-degree students at prestigious institutions—recognize that every student is unique and take a holistic one-on-one approach to their applications. By honing in on the student's individual strengths, personal qualities, and professional goals, our experts are able to guide them into crafting well-written and compelling personal statements, strengthening their resumes and application materials, and thoroughly prepping them for the highly-sought interview round.

It's no mystery that medical school admissions are a marathon, a lengthy, grueling, and serious commitment, and this reality informs our long-term approach at Moon Prep in the relationships we build with our students and their families. These relationships can often span several years, and our success rates have brought us a high referral rate among siblings and other highly-qualified candidates. We are fortunate to work with some of the most elite students in their academic circles, where they excel in their courses, exams, and extracurricular activities. Our number one priority lies in serving them and their families who support them. We understand their relentless focus on securing top-notch grades and high scores for their applications, and we build on this foundation to help them secure research opportunities, medical internships, leadership experience, and other invaluable insights.

One key aspect of this versatility is their success during the crucial series of multiple mini-interviews, an interview process unique to medical admissions. These interviews give admission committees a holistic view of the applicants, allowing them to learn more about their character traits, observe their communication skills, assess their thought processes, and gauge their capacity for teamwork, collaboration, and professionalism.

As we help our students take that monumental next step into the world of medicine, we marvel every year at their incredible transformations into rising leaders and outstanding young citizens, an impressive cohort we know will go on to serve their communities and remind us of our shared humanity. This is why we have such a fantastic and rewarding job at Moon Prep: we are polishing gemstones and preparing these young people for bright futures. And this book is one more part of that never-ending guidance and support, giving us the opportunity to share our wealth of experience and insights into proven strategies that secure admission at some of the most competitive medical schools. Our students—and many others around the world—need a more complete understanding of not only the academic, leadership, and essay requirements for admissions success, but equally important, the nuanced best practices that will help them stand out for the admissions committee during the MMI process.

Kristen Moon

— Kristen Moon, MBA
Founder & CEO, Moon Prep
www.moonprep.com

1

INTRODUCTION TO THE MMI

When you consider the health and well-being of the individuals in our society—our families, our loved ones—there's arguably nothing more important than quality medical care.

For those called to a career in medicine, your goals are clear: Help people live better and healthier lives, support the sick and injured in their most trying times, provide trusted medical guidance to your patients—guidance that's built on years of study, knowledge, training, and experience—and apply it to challenging, real-life situations.

It's a noble profession because it's so critical to our daily lives.

But to obtain this career, you must first graduate from a respected medical school program. You need to earn professional credentials from an accredited and established institution to give patients confidence in your abilities to heal them.

For those making this decision when still in high

school, direct medical programs [BS/MD and BS/DO] offer the clearest path to making your dream and life goals a reality. For those on the traditional path to medicine, you want to know that your time in medical school has prepared you with the real-world skills you'll need.

With growing interest in healthcare careers, medical school acceptance is coveted among those pursuing higher education. In fact, admission to some of the country's best programs has become increasingly selective. Acceptance rates at these programs can be as low as 1% or less.

Why? Because they can be.

Medical school applicants regularly apply with comprehensive dossiers filled with stellar high school grades (with matching [GPA] grade point averages), especially in their science and math classes; a strong record of extracurricular activities, including student leadership, musical study, sports participation, etc.; a record of community and volunteer work; strong standardized test scores; and more.

Between high expectations of being well-rounded, the fierce application process, and competitiveness, medical school acceptances are often viewed as a badge of honor. The privilege of holding a position as a medical student is an emblem of perseverance and dedication to excellence.

What can BS/MD and pre-med students do to have a competitive edge in the application process?

Simple… Be fully prepared.

The more you understand the entire process of medical school and BS/MD admissions can prevent any surprise requirements along the way. Adequate preparation will help you appropriately frame your application and put forth a strong demonstration of your candidacy to admissions offices. Once admission officers have determined a pool of qualified individuals, they need to narrow down their list of potential candidates for a limited number of seats. It takes more than a high GPA, glowing references, a thoughtful personal statement, and a stellar transcript to earn an acceptance letter.

Enter the critical interview process.

This process typically consists of two types of interviews: standard and the Multiple Mini Interview [MMI]. In addition to academic rigor, the admissions counselors and committees are looking for prospective students with strong communication skills and empathy to become a physician. Interviews reveal much more about a candidate's interpersonal skills, maturity, motivation, and interest in being a physician, as well as a sense of their moral and ethical fabric. Because of this, medical school admissions departments rely heavily on the interview process to screen their candidates. Many institutions employ the MMI format, with its short problem-based stations, which deliver this vital information to reviewers in an efficient way.

Traditionally, the interview process at most medical schools and BS/MD (direct medical programs) was a simple one-on-one meeting with an admissions officer reviewing the same boilerplate questions with each applicant. Of course, it's a useful tool, so you can expect to still take part in a standard or traditional interview, even if it is more limited.

Here's what the traditional interview process looks like:

You step into a room, meet the interviewer, and have a seat. After exchanging a couple of pleasantries, these are likely the four most common questions you'll encounter in traditional medical school interviews:

- Tell me about yourself
- Why do you want to be a doctor?
- Why have you chosen our institution to continue your studies?
- What are your strengths and weaknesses?

Read those again, and this time, give yourself at least a few minutes to plan your answers. Optimally, you'd say each answer out loud to hear exactly what it would sound like in conversation. (Practice with a friend or record yourself on your phone if that makes the process feel more time-based. Ask each question as the admissions committee and then record your answers.) As you listen back, you'll be able to tell how articulate and natural you sound answering these interview questions.

Prep Tip: If this standard interview set is hard for you at this stage, write lists that answer each question in a variety of ways. Be honest... Why DO you want to be a doctor? You could probably fill an entire page that would include factors like making a difference in the world and your community, honor/prestige, respect from family/peers, etc. Force yourself to have ten answers for each question —even if it requires some research on your part — and then narrow your answers down to the best and most accurate response.

These standard questions are still valuable and enlightening for admissions committees, but, as you can see, they are quite limiting as well. Why? The medical schools know very well that students often rehearse a set of canned responses to questions like these and practice them over and over with counselors, coaches, and family members. However, a series of interviews on various topics provide more opportunities to learn about your values and integrity.

The MMI, Multiple Mini Interviews, which originated at McMaster University in Hamilton, Ontario, Canada, but wasn't introduced in the United States until 2008, fills this role. Each year, it expands to more and more medical schools. (see appendix for participating schools). Its dynamic interview process allows several evaluators to meet with a medical school's best candidates and listen to them speak, reason, deal with role-playing scenarios, respond to ethical questions, and more. For our BS/MD students, the overall interview format will be the same as it is for medical school students. However, BS/MD students will encounter different types of questions than what med students might expect. More information on the question types can be found in Chapter Four.

Next, let's talk about how this book can help you in the MMI.

2

HOW THIS BOOK WILL HELP
YOU PREPARE

O f course, the actual format and structure of the interviews vary by institution — number of stations and evaluators, breaks, note-taking rules during scenarios, etc. But if they have invited you to an interview—whether standard or MMI—congratulations! You are one step closer to medical school and on the path to your life as a physician.

If you haven't been invited to an MMI (multiple mini interviews) yet, this book will help you use your application time more efficiently. This project was designed to help you prepare for the MMI because it can be your key to medical school admission, either through the BS/MD or the traditional route. And because the MMI process is partly shrouded in secrecy and confidentiality, some widespread assumptions about the MMI process by applicants, parents, and guidance counselors are incorrect and can impede your prep strategy.

This book collects best practices about the MMI, discusses a preparation and response strategy, and points

KRISTEN MOON

you in the direction of the work you need to complete before you attend your first applicant MMI. Along the way, the book will help dispel myths about the MMI that may harm your chances of a positive outcome.

The general categories of MMI evaluations depend on the institution, but applicants can expect these types of questions:

- Stations related to complex ethical dilemmas
- Stations with acting or role-playing scenarios (if it is a virtual interview, you will likely not have role-playing scenario questions)
- Stations focused almost entirely on critical thinking
- Stations that explore your knowledge and understanding of the United States healthcare system in its current state
- Stations that may require a written response of some sort, whether that's informative, creative, or persuasive (if it is a virtual interview, you will likely not have written response questions)
- Stations that explore your past behaviors or situation-specific judgment or decisions. Has your response changed over time because of your growth, experiences, maturity, or simply access to new information, and how is your ability to reflect on those events in your past?
- Stations that touch on the typical traditional interview questions, often with some variations

COMMON MISCONCEPTIONS ABOUT THE MMI

One such myth is that you cannot prepare yourself in advance for the MMI. It's not true. While it's impossible to know which questions will be asked during your interview, as you work through the material presented here, you'll be prepared to develop strong responses to any type of questions on interview day. Understanding the utility of these interviews to the overall admissions process can help you present yourself in the best possible light.

It's never too early (or late) to review this material. It should aid in any preparation you undertake and will give you time to research topics you might feel less prepared to discuss. One such example is the state of the U.S. healthcare system and how you would improve upon these issues. Although science and math may seem disproportionately more important, medical school programs expect you to have some articulate commentary on its structure, including Medicaid and Medicare. For medical school applicants who discover this requirement early, you'll have plenty of time to do the relevant research.

There is also the misconception that there are no wrong answers to MMI questions. Again, this is not true. There are several responses to individual and collaborative situations that would clearly display to the evaluators that you are not of the right temperament for the medical profession.

Some applicants think the MMI process is less important because the evaluators are often not medical school faculty or admissions personnel. Again, this is not true. Every MMI evaluator will write a score based on your

KRISTEN MOON

performance in a mini-interview regardless of whether they are faculty, current medical students, retired health-care professionals, campus staff, or members of the community. MMIs are closed file interviews, meaning the interviewers know nothing about you besides what they see in the interview. Their evaluations from these six to ten stations carry weight in your acceptance decision.

Although the MMI does not require previous knowl-edge of medical procedures, basic anatomy or health, or diagnoses, it still evaluates interpersonal and intraper-sonal skills that are highly regarded by medical profes-sionals. Admissions committees across the entire spectrum of medical schools have confirmed how central these interviews are to their decision-making process.

The MMI was introduced as another way to evaluate students on a level that reveals important qualities medical professionals need, like communication, leader-ship, teamwork, empathy, problem-solving, cultural awareness, conflict resolution skills, robust ethics, informed public health awareness, and more.

Some applicants like the MMI process interviews; they might find MMI seemingly more fair, somewhat enjoyable, and more intuitive than standard interviews. With a couple of minutes to read the scenario and/or prompt before entering the classroom, office, partition, or virtual meeting room, it's the ultimate test of staying focused on only what is truly at hand. And because these do not test your medical knowledge, it's a much more comprehensive tool to assess your empathy, resilience, communication, and other "soft skills."

Of course, if it works organically during these scenar-ios, you're free to include information about your experi-ences, especially if it reveals to the evaluator some part of your decision-making process. Your answers and responses to the challenge scenarios will then have professionalism mixed with some context and authenticity.

Medical school applicants might prefer the MMI process because it gives them a chance to display their full range of preparation as young people embarking on a path towards medicine: their skills, range of individualized experiences, empathy and compassion, emotional intelligence, and more. While a transcript or letter of reference demonstrates a candidate's abilities to succeed in medical school, MMI reveals more about the character of the student and how they react under pressure.

Next up, let's talk strategy.

3

MMI STRATEGY DISCUSSION

Expect that many institutions you apply to may use either the MMI-only interview or a hybrid format of MMI combined with traditional one-on-one interviews. When you get the interview request, it will detail what type of interview you can expect, so there are no surprises. However, it's in your best interest to be fully prepared for both types. Beyond learning about the process, expectations, and utility of the MMI in medical school admissions, there are specific strategies that will help you as you take part in your series of six to ten mini-interviews.

Here are examples of some of the homework you can do before any medical school interview:

- Outline examples of accomplishments in your life that were reached because of your ability to work effectively on a team toward a common goal. Be prepared to explain each example clearly and succinctly.

- If you're confronted by a tough problem, do you have several critical thinking tools to work toward a solution? Consider your strengths and weaknesses when it comes to problem-solving.
- If you encounter complex social, family, domestic, and ethical issues, do you have the empathy and compassion to discuss these in both a supportive and professional manner? Go through and create a list of hot-button topics and evaluate where you stand on each — both in your ethical core and your rational sense of a physician's role in those issues. Some of these hot-button topics could include: cross-cultural issues and diverse beliefs, abortions and birth control, HIV and AIDs, Do Not Resuscitate orders, end-of-life issues, genetics, treatment refusal, public health ethics, and much more.
- Overall, how well versed are you on the touchstone ethical issues in our society, especially those that intersect with the modern health care system? You should be prepared to speak on a range of topics in and around medicine, healthcare, social issues, and more. A well-rounded medical student is an important foundation for a well-rounded doctor who is a pillar of their community, not just their medical practice. Make another list here of topics that you need to work on during your preparations.

REMEMBER YOUR COMMUNICATION SKILLS ARE ALWAYS ON DISPLAY

As you contemplate a career in medicine and the process of medical school admissions, reflect on your overall communication skills. Do you consider yourself capable of clearly expressing yourself in any situation? Can you express your morals, ethical core, and empathetic nature, as well as complex science, math, and other topics of a more technical nature?

Communication skills and non-verbal skills like teamwork, self-awareness, maturity, empathy, and critical thinking are difficult to assess with standardized testing, so they are at the core of what's being evaluated with the MMI. Knowing this, how can you possibly sharpen your communication skills in the time you have before these interviews?

Simple... practice. But before we practice, let's try to understand the full scope of what's being assessed. As we work on our communication skills, we will also supplement your grasp of high-yield content.

One common topic to review is the general topic of ethics, especially as it relates to the healthcare system, to practice articulating your views on complex issues.

But what if you're tired, nervous, or feeling overwhelmed on the day of the MMIs? How can you approach these types of challenges? Listen closely to the scenario at hand, take a stance on an ethical issue, and be prepared to defend it. Even if your evaluator disagrees with you, it is important to realize that they are trying to gauge your understanding and ability to develop and articulate important concepts. Like in a debate club, they want to see if you can take a side in a polarizing debate

KRISTEN MOON

and clearly explain your perspective, even when confronted with an opposing viewpoint. More importantly, can you do this while maintaining your composure? One of the best ways to practice is recording yourself discussing a specific topic for a set amount of time. As you review your recording, watch carefully to see if you were clear and logical as you articulated your point of view.

While each station will typically last about 8-10 minutes, do not use all of your allotted time in the station on your initial response. It is often a good strategy to save a few minutes at the end of your response to answer any follow-up questions from the interviewer.

OTHER STRATEGIC CHOICES YOU CAN MAKE DURING YOUR MMI

Listening is a skill that almost cannot be overstated.

Can you consistently listen closely to all the participants, evaluators, and scenarios? Although it's unlikely that they designed the MMI formats with trick questions, you can expect that attention to detail is the key to fully understanding what is being asked of you. By listening closely, you are also displaying a key skill for physicians or any medical professional who must listen to all patients and family members closely and without making assumptions about what is being communicated.

- Do you pay close attention to the details of each scenario and parse what you're hearing so you can evaluate both the content and what isn't being said?

MOON PREP'S GUIDE TO MMI

- Do your responses display your open mind and willingness to learn?
- Do you have a wide enough set of experiences to back up your ideas, thoughts, etc.?
- Are you open to other perspectives, but still able to explain your convictions?
- Can you display in your answers that you don't overstep established boundaries and don't work outside established laws and regulations? Do you understand the limitations of your practice as a medical doctor in our society? While you need to understand how to work around the current system, medical schools still like for you to contemplate ways for you to improve the system. However, you need to present it in a practical way with the understanding that one person alone cannot change a systemic issue. For example, you can talk about how you could collaborate with like-minded peers to advocate for issues or help change policies.
- Can you be direct and not intentionally avoid any difficult aspects of the scenarios which are likely to be scored?

Recovery from conflicts and difficulties is a skill every medical professional needs. And many of these scenario-based interviews are uniquely designed to test this. Consider your ability to be challenged, thrown, or rattled in one MMI setup, and then leave that experience behind and move on to the next station with a clear and open mind. Each station is a fresh, new interview. Can you stay completely focused on the task at hand and not get caught up reflecting, rethinking, and regretting things you said or didn't say in your previous scenarios? Can you compartmentalize your emotions and reset your critical listening and critical thinking skills in the context of any situational difficulties? We'd all agree that physicians need these skills, and the MMI offers a format that provides the opportunity for a medical school to evaluate you.

A common topic that medical school applicants struggle with during MMI sessions is questions related to legal matters. Most problematic among those are scenarios specifically dealing with any medical treatments related to a life-threatening situation or in the treatment of minors.

As an applicant, you are not expected to know all the current medical laws. Instead, what is assessed and judged during the interview process is your critical thinking on these topics and related matters. For BS/MD students especially, you will likely not be judged on your knowledge of medical laws at all, but instead, be placed in scenarios that solely judge your critical thinking. For all MMI students, as you display your ability to think through these cases logically, your evaluators will respond with positive feedback on their rating forms.

So here's a starting point for all applicants: the primary overarching goal for physicians specifically is, of course, to provide judgment in the best interest of the patient. Remembering this will often guide you while you make decisions that are fraught with complex legal or moral implications.

HOW TO APPROACH MMI QUESTIONS

When you enter the interview room, you typically have two minutes to read the MMI prompt, take notes (if allowed), and formulate your strategy. This time should be used wisely to ensure you are looking at the issue from multiple perspectives.

In these two minutes, you should not only be thinking about what you are reading but what is unsaid in the prompt. Think about what questions pop up as you read the prompt. This will help direct your thoughts. Take this scenario as an example:

A 13-year-old patient walks into your clinic with her parents. When her parents leave the room for the exam, she reveals that she has been having unprotected sex and would like to go on birth control. She also says that if you tell her parents about her request, she will deny it and find another way to get the pills. How do you handle the situation?

Before you start thinking about the approach, think about what you know and what you don't know:

- Can you treat her the same as an adult? Or should you inform her patients? What are the laws in your state?
- With what frequency is she having unprotected sex, and how many partners?
- Has she been tested for STIs?
- Does she understand the risks of unprotected sex or taking drugs that haven't been prescribed to her?

Thinking about the questions that you have will help

you figure out the right path to follow. As you formulate the response, while you do want to consider all the information and possibilities, you *must* take a stance. While you might show great insight into your understanding of whether or not a 13-year-old patient should be treated as an adult, if you don't actually state *how* you would treat her as a patient, then you aren't using your time wisely.

Often for MMI questions, there is no one right answer—your scenario could unfold in a number of certain ways, depending on some of the answers to the questions that you asked yourself originally. Medical schools know that you may not know all of the treatment protocols, so this will not be held against you. Rather, they are evaluating you on your ability to think logically and develop a plan based on different outcomes that can occur in the given scenario. By addressing those different avenues out loud to your interviewer, you showcase your abilities to be flexible, read the situation, and anticipate different outcomes. Ultimately, many MMI questions will have you address complex questions, but you must take a stance by showcasing your thought process with a clear answer.

URGENT MEDICAL TREATMENT IN LIFE-THREATENING SITUATIONS

The work of medical professionals, while often routine and focused on preventative care, sometimes includes dealing with life-threatening situations. Patients can live or die based on the decisions made in a hospital or ER, or by any medical care team.

But you will not be making these decisions alone or without the experience of increased patient-care responsibilities. Over time, this becomes a key skill for young physicians: the ability to make these decisions under pressure and when a patient's life is on the line.

In a complicated situation involving life-threatening treatment, a doctor must determine whether the patient can make an informed decision. It's also possible that another person has a POA (power of attorney) and the hospital staff must try to find that out. Beyond that, the next of kin, possibly the spouse or legal partner, parents, siblings, or close friends, can also play a role.

Remember the guiding principle here: if no one can be reached to help decide or weigh in on the care, the doctor's strategy is obvious. Do everything within your power to save the patient.

However, BS/MD students will not be expected to answer questions because they will have limited exposure to working and volunteering in the healthcare field. BS/MD students will likely not encounter questions that test their knowledge of what medical treatment to give in certain situations.

MEDICAL CARE ISSUES WHILE TREATING MINORS

Doctors are always expected to treat minors (children under age 18) in all life-threatening situations, regardless of parental consent.

Think of it this way. Suppose a critical, time-sensitive medical procedure or surgery could save a child's life and the parents and guardians are unreachable. In that case, it does not make any legal, moral, or professional sense to wait to receive confirmation to approve medical intervention. As expected, parents and guardians would typically

KRISTEN MOON

want the medical establishment to do everything within their power to save the child, even if they weren't contacted.

Alternatively, if you have a life-saving treatment available for a minor, but the parent does not consent to treatment, you have a legal obligation to still perform the treatment. In these types of cases, you can get a court order. The bottom line is that you will always treat minors in life-threatening conditions. However, if the minor is not in a life-threatening condition, then parents still have the right to refuse treatment, and your duty as the physician is to educate the family on the risks and benefits and respect their autonomy.

Furthermore, physicians and other medical professionals are expected to maintain patient confidentiality in all matters dealing with drug use, mental health, and sexual health. Let this be your guide as you consider the most complex and demanding MMI scenarios. Also, remember that minors who are emancipated and/or pregnant can legally make their own legal decisions.

Again, BS/MD students will likely not encounter scenarios or prompts that require more advanced knowledge on the nuances of handling patient care, especially for minors.

ETHICAL GUIDANCE

Because MMI questions are purposely vague, make sure you fully understand the parameters of any ethical or moral issue and gather more information. You are allowed to ask your interviewer qualifying questions if you need more specific information. Weigh the risks and benefits in any complex medical situation, both with and without treatment, and consider all real-life consequences. Whenever you can, provide a solution—even if it's just a referral to another resource that can provide more information to your patient.

This approach demonstrates your ability to create a clear plan that builds trust with patients. It also provides them with facts, information, and professional advice, while allowing them to make their own decisions. It is not your place to decide your patient's medical treatments, but rather to support them through education. However, if there is a legal issue, you may be called to take a stance in that scenario.

As you answer ethical dilemmas, make sure to consider whether any ethical pillar has been breached:

- Autonomy — a patient has the freedom to make decisions regarding their healthcare procedures free of coercion or coaxing. To make an informed decision, a patient should understand the risks and benefits of the treatment.
- Beneficence — a doctor acts with the intention of doing good for the patient involved.
- Social justice —this principle ensures fairness; physicians must decide if the action is compatible with the law, and the patient's rights, and if it is fair and balanced to all.
- Non-maleficence —this idea requires that the treatment does not harm the patient or others. This requires physicians to operate under the assumption that they are either doing no harm or minimizing harm for the greater good.

Think about these two ethical challenge conflicts:

- Some workers under your supervision are cutting corners that are, in part, detrimental to clients, customers, etc. Of these employees, one is the daughter of a company board member. How would you deal with this? Would your job security concerns override your ethical core and morality in this situation?
- What if your position as a medical administrator gave you early access to critical life-saving medicine or vaccines? If you're not in any increased danger working in an office without patient contact, would you delay your access to the treatment or immunization, especially during a serious outbreak where many others more critically needed the protection?

While the answers to these questions might seem obvious, can you explain them in your own words, incorporating the principles of the ethical pills into your approach to these dilemmas?

As you work through ethical dilemma questions, remember you can appeal to a higher authority like the law or management in the workplace. These structures can help us approach the questions and navigate the gray waters that these dilemmas present. However, if presented with a challenging ethical situation, we want to explore other options besides management. You shouldn't be solely relying on higher authorities in your answer, but you can use them whenever the situation calls for it.

As a physician, you will treat patients of a different cultural or religious background than you. Cultural competence will be a trait that the interviewers evaluate during the interview. While you aren't expected to understand the nuances of every religion or culture, you should display cultural awareness in your response to form a competent response.

Expect questions like these across a broad spectrum of categories, which require you to expand on your morals and ethics. Ahead, you'll find two chapters of MMI-style sample questions, each followed by a brief discussion of strategy, complexity, prep advice, and more.

4

SAMPLE MMI QUESTIONS FOR BS/MD AND MEDICAL SCHOOL STUDENTS, PART ONE

Here is a range of unique MMI-style questions extrapolated from medical school admissions departments and based on feedback from successful candidates. After the sample questions, there are brief discussions of the skills, abilities, and challenges likely being assessed, as well as some commentary you can use to plan your own strategic approach to answer them. While you may not encounter these exact questions during your interview, broadly preparing with questions like these will help you tackle the same sorts of challenges and illuminate the same character traits for the evaluators.

These questions could be asked at both BS/MD and medical school interviews.

1. Someone very close to you has chosen an alternative medicine treatment for a serious illness. Would you discuss this with them?

Traditional medicine has always been challenged and

KRISTEN MOON

supported by a world of alternative treatments, some of which have long cultural traditions. The first part of this challenge is the moral and ethical choice you'd make on whether to initiate a conversation on mainstream versus alternative treatments, knowing the possible difficult discussion you might have with someone who has already decided. You want to understand how they learned about this choice and why they chose this specific therapy. This question also speaks to your ability to be supportive of a patient's choices but also offers to help them realize a range of possible effective treatments available in traditional medicine, even if they're already convinced by their decision.

The challenge is to be fully sensitive to the patient's choices and give them the autonomy to make those choices, but also give them other options and information based on your experience so they can make a better informed medical decision.

You want to initiate the conversation in this order:

- come from a place of understanding
- introduce traditional therapy
- discuss risk and benefits of alternative medicine and traditional medicine
- allow them to make their choice

2. Discuss your experience with an extreme stress situation and how you dealt with it. (Follow up: What would you do differently now — if anything — if you faced the same situation?)

Everyone deals with stress in their lives. But while others might casually think about the stress and pressures from a past event, they rarely have to recount the story of those events to others.

28

The challenge here is to concisely discuss your past stressors and your ability to contextualize the way you dealt with them at the moment. Additionally, you're given a chance to reflect on how you might process the same experiences now, which speaks to your maturity and growth. It also speaks to your candor, your ability to handle life's most difficult situations, and your ability to express yourself even when discussing something very painful or trying in your life.

Note: If there is another person involved in this stressful situation, tread carefully when recounting your story and be sure to not place blame entirely on the other person. A good way to prevent yourself from sounding accusatory is to start with "I felt...", as opposed to "John wronged by doing ....".

3. If we asked your friends and family to describe you, what would they say? (Follow up: What do you think is the most important quality for a doctor to have?)

Of course, friends and family have a bias when it comes to you. That's understood.

This question and similar ones provide a chance for you to reflect on yourself as a person in your community, in your family unit, and among friends in your school or neighborhood. This could also be a way to bring up extracurricular activities if they help define your character.

Note: This question could also be framed as "If we asked your peers, teachers, professors, etc, to describe you, what would they say?" Your response could be very similar to the previous question, but you'll want to tailor your examples to be from a more academic setting. This challenge is more about what you can contextualize beyond what they say and provides another window into your maturity and self-awareness. It's also an opportunity to suggest areas in your life and study that your mentors might identify as areas of improvement for you.

4. Discuss the last book you read. What did you get from it?

Medical schools often appreciate candidates who have hobbies and are well-read. Here's your chance to display your current reading habits — a relatively simple and proven way to better yourself. Plan to discuss your latest discretionary reading choice and any specific lessons you garnered from that reading.

What often trips students up with these types of questions is they give an answer based on what they think the interviewer wants to hear. You might think that mentioning medical textbooks or science or math prep books might show that you're a diligent student attempting to fill in any deficiencies in your current understanding of difficult science courses. However, answering this way would be a missed opportunity if you have another current read that reveals something about your interests outside of medicine.

Note: This question could also be asked as "Describe your favorite film. (Follow up: Why do you love it and what lessons can you learn from it about life, storytelling, etc?)."

Questions like this, while seemingly simple on the surface, reveal a lot about your character, your worldview, and more. You should be honest about a movie or film that has affected you and not simply choose something random because you think it will make you sound smarter. Be prepared to explain your rationale for your preferences. Be ready to unpack what it is about the creative work that speaks to you (i.e., relatable characters, an aligned vision of the future, the heroic lead character(s), touching story, powerful life lessons, etc.).

5. In your opinion, what is the primary responsibility of a doctor?

There are so many possible answers to this question; because of that, some applicants assume they can't go wrong with any response. Like many informed opinion-based challenges, however, many things are being assessed here as you answer.

This is your chance as a medical school applicant to reflect on the overall job of a physician and the range of responsibilities that come with that position. After you've identified them, you must choose one as being the primary responsibility and then clearly articulate why you chose it. Supplement your answer with insight, or more ideally, an example pulled from your medical shadowing and volunteer experience. This type of question has a range of appropriate answers, so a large part of what is being evaluated here is your ability to support your opinion clearly and concisely.

6. Your close friend misses work or college classes and often smells of alcohol. Next time you see them, what do you do?

This is a challenge to showcase your interpersonal and conflict resolution skills. It raises the question of not only how you would approach an issue like this but also whether you would choose to intervene at all. While this is not an issue of patient care, it is about how you would demonstrate your care and concern for a close friend or associate. It's also a model for how you might approach a difficult conversation. This MMI question focuses on your basic communication skills, especially in a potentially emotional situation.

KRISTEN MOON

If a scenario like this is played out with another person in the role of your close friend, you'll have to display to the evaluator how you would handle both the initial conflict and the potential range of emotions that may follow when you broach this topic: denial, anger, shame, push back, defensiveness, and more.

7. How would you describe your sensitivity when it comes to the needs of others? Give a recent example.

This is the sort of MMI question that could be either easy or quite difficult to answer. Here's an opportunity to display your capacity to be caring and empathetic towards others as you aspire to understand their wants and needs. You'll be required to think on your feet to come up with authentic examples from your own life. Remember that the work that medical professionals do necessitates genuine care for their patients. As you describe your sensitivity and explain it in a way that shows compassion for others, you demonstrate that you have the empathy and engagement required to be an effective physician.

8. If you're accepted into a medical school program, what do you think your greatest challenge will be?

For this question, there is a range of hurdles to consider: an intense workload, specialized coursework, communication challenges, leadership responsibilities, displaying grace under pressure, collaborating with peers, responding well to criticism, and more.

If you listen closely to what's being asked, however, you'll see that you'll need to reflect on what you think your greatest challenge will be. In some ways, it's a variant of the strengths and weaknesses question that fills most standard interviews, but with a specific emphasis on the obstacles you'll face in medical school. Whether you think the science curriculum will be hard, the teamwork, etc... anything you say is a very revealing answer about your preparation to enter their program. But knowing yourself well enough to see the challenges far in advance—and being open and honest about them—is a very mature display of your confidence and self-awareness as a young person. As you answer this question, make sure to be specific and talk about not only why this particular challenge, but also how you might overcome the challenge.

9. If it was your responsibility to tell a terminally ill cancer patient that he/she has only a few weeks to live, how would you say it? (Follow up: Have you ever had to deliver bad news to anyone, and what did you learn from that experience?)

In this type of either direct question or role-playing exercise, you will need to seriously consider how you would deliver this news, including how you would set the scene for delivering the news. What exact words would you choose, and why? As you consider your response to this question, think about the ethical pillars of medicine and how that might guide you in your response. Based on your maturity and life experiences combined with ethics, morality, and empathy, how would you want to be told if you were the patient? Remember that this question focuses not on the medical details of the diagnosis but rather on the empathy and sensitivity you display in your patient interaction.

For the follow-up, you likely wouldn't have had to deliver news on a similar scale, but try to think of an example of a time that you had to give harsh feedback or bad news. By sharing how you handled a similar situation, the interviewers can start to picture what type of

KRISTEN MOON

physician you'll be when you're forced to deliver an unwelcome diagnosis.

10. Describe a current role model in your life, not necessarily related to the medical field.

With this question, you can talk about any person or mentor you look up to in your life. Because the key word here is "describe," you have to explain, honestly and compellingly, how this person fulfills a role as someone you respect and aspire to be like in your life, your career, and growth as an individual.

Be careful with answers that sound corny, insincere, or hackneyed. It's better not to choose a historical figure but instead someone you know in real life, as this would allow you to recount personal experiences and interactions that have specifically inspired you.

If you don't have a specific role model who comes to mind, consider people (both living and dead) who have helped you understand valuable life lessons, whether connected to your pursuit of medicine or not. You can then reflect on what it would be like to find a mentor or role model in the future. Additionally, with enough reading across an array of disciplines, you'll likely find someone who you'd consider a role model for your current stage in life.

11. Considering the current state of the healthcare system in the United States, what do you consider to be the top two to three issues which reduce its efficiency?

As a future physician, it's important to be well-informed about our modern healthcare system, admiring its benefits while still being realistically unsatisfied with its shortcomings. The challenge here is speaking your mind, but also holding your optimism for a field to which you plan to devote your life and career.

This type of overall policy question is common in many medical schools because it reveals your understanding of the healthcare system as a whole, both in the areas that function well and the parts mired in bureaucracies, inefficiencies, poor outcomes, and worse. It's not a test to see how much you know about health care laws or the minutiae of Medicare and Medicaid, but more so a challenge to see if you have any real context about the field you're hoping to enter and if you can speak intelligently about its issues and drawbacks.

Stay constructive and utilize your exceptional communication skills to not only share the changes you'd like to see but also your intentions to help change the profession in your individualized way.

12. If you were challenged by a medical school professor on your ability to handle the workload and coursework required in their program, what would you say?

This question speaks to an applicant's realistic outlook on the coursework and study workloads required in a medical school program. Take this opportunity to describe how you have the background, experience, drive, work ethic, and time management skills to handle the challenges ahead. Elevate your answer by sharing with your evaluator specific examples of your ability to handle mountains of responsibilities.

For in-person interviews, you might also encounter this as a role-playing scenario opposite a professor who has some opinions about your capabilities. While this sort of station may be initially intimidating, it also allows a chance for you to show how you would handle a professional conflict. With that, it's important to maintain your composure and describe your skills with respect. Your

KRISTEN MOON

response should be objective, level-headed, and logical without sounding defensive.

13. What drives you to want to become a doctor, and what specialties are you most interested in?

Here's a common question in traditional interviews that allows the evaluator to hear your thoughts about medical specialties and your future. This question speaks to your motivations to enter the medical field and your ability to articulate your intentions to an evaluator. The specialty research shows your breadth of understanding of the profession and the chance to show your interests and passions in your career planning.

Remember, you aren't committing to a certain specialty in the interview; they just want to learn more about what motivates you to enter the field and where your interests are right now. It's also okay if you aren't certain yet—state a few specialties you'd like to explore further and why. You can also express your excitement and anticipation of learning more about these fields as you continue your medical education.

14. If you see an accident victim while driving, would you stop and help?

Expect ethical questions like these in the MMI process. The answers are enlightening for the evaluators because they speak to your mindset and indicate any fears you may have about being a physician. Here's another chance to display your problem-solving skills combined with your core ethical and moral standards. Would you help? If not, why not? It's a balance between doing what's right and wrong versus understanding the liability that medical professionals face in their work.

15. Where do you plan to practice medicine? What various locations have you considered and why?

MOON PREP'S GUIDE TO MMI

Here's a chance to show how thoughtful and focused you are about your career plans and outline your career interests. What patient populations are you passionate about working with? Have you considered specific urban, suburban, and/or rural areas for your medical practice? Would you prefer to be a member of an innovative team at a state-of-the-art urban hospital group, or would you choose to fill a much-needed medical position in an underserved rural community? Would you work inside the United States, or would you consider a post in another country; if so, where and why would you be drawn to practice medicine there? Be prepared to support your answer, whatever it may be, with insight and examples, if possible.

16. If a magician, genie, or wizard granted you three wishes in your life or career, what would they be?

While this seems like a light and fun question, your answer reveals a lot about your character, aspirations, hopes and dreams, and even general worldview. Knowing that it's a loaded question shouldn't keep you from answering honestly; it's just another example of a medical mini-interview challenge where you have to consider the ramifications of what you're saying.

If your wishes are broad-based, it can give a sense of your real self-awareness. If all your answers are about medicine, medical school, and your career aspirations, you're signaling to the evaluators that you're either very ambitious (not necessarily a bad thing), or you're incorrectly assuming that those are the answers that they most want to hear, which is not always the case. A range of solid, thoughtful answers, medically relevant or otherwise, will do well at this type of station.

17. How would you describe the difference between empathy and compassion?

This is not a simple semantics question about the meaning of these words. It's a chance for you to reveal something to the evaluator about your moral and ethical core. In a broad question like this, it helps to give examples from your personal experiences that indicate that you truly understand the differences.

18. Do you consider yourself adaptable? Give an example. (Follow up: Do you believe you'll become more or less adaptable as your career evolves?)

This is another deep and revealing question about your self-awareness. Adaptability, mutability, and your overall willingness to change and develop are critical to your growth as a physician. An understanding of your current level of adaptability, supported by concrete examples, is necessary.

The follow-up question is also challenging because it implies that with experience and career maturity, there is potential for that adaptability to change. Regardless of your answer, don't treat this as a binary query and only say "yes" or "no." Have some logic behind your response and explain your thought process to the evaluator.

19. How is integrity meaningful to you? Give examples.

Of course, living a life led by honor with a solid ethical core is something most people would endorse. The challenge here is to provide specific examples of how it's meaningful specifically to you. Where has your word, the promises you or others have made, or your moral compass displayed its central meaning in your life?

This MMI question could be answered in a variety of ways; recounting a situation where you were wronged by a person without integrity or sharing your insight into

MOON PREP'S GUIDE TO MMI

how integrity can define your place in the world are two possible examples of how to go about this station. As is the case with all MMI questions, be sure to adequately describe your thoughts behind your answer.

20. If you were not working in the field of medicine, what would you do and why?

For some students, this question rattles them. Do these institutions really want to hear about the fall-back plan for candidates who don't ever get accepted to medical school? Are they trying to evaluate how much confidence you have in your first choice of medicine versus any alternative career goal?

Although it feels like a trick question to be answered with an 'all or nothing' response, it reveals maturity, self-awareness, and more to discuss another field of interest. If there is a common skill-set overlapping your choices, then there's no conflict. For example, a young medical school student who aspires to be a surgeon but who could also envision a career as a concert violinist because of the precision in their hands, attention to detail, and the physical demands of concentration, is not a slight against a career in medicine.

It is also important to remember that part of the interview is seeing how you respond to intentionally difficult questions. If you are unsure of how to answer, do not be afraid to take a few seconds to center yourself and collect your thoughts. Your evaluator will better appreciate a slow and thoughtful answer than they would a quick but rambled response.

21. If you were tasked with fixing homelessness, what would you do?

This is an ethical, moral, and big-picture perspective question that shows your ability to think on your feet and unpack your ideas in real time. This is also an opportunity for the evaluators to openly disagree with you to see how you respond to healthy debate and/or conflict. Take all questions like this seriously, even if you struggle to come up with an answer. Again, what's useful for the MMI team is to hear your problem-solving process, so even if you are unsure, walking through a few ideas of what you might do could be useful in revealing your skills at working towards a solution.

22. If a patient you're treating tells you they want to die, what would you do?

Patients are often faced with the stress of their own mortality while also being saddled with catastrophic illness, chronic pain, severe loss of quality of life, and more. In addition, they are often under extreme personal stress secondary to their medical challenges spilling over into their family lives with marital and parental responsibilities, financial concerns (i.e., insurance), job issues, and more.

This is another ethical and moral question you could face as a professional physician. As you formulate your response, think of the ethical pillars of medicine. Whether this is simply a question or revealed to you through a role-playing exercise, the evaluators want to hear the exact steps you would take and in what order. To prepare for this, you must consider the limits of your professional patient care options and the potential need for you to refer your patients for additional counseling with a psychologist, psychiatrist, or social worker.

23. Do you believe it's ethical for doctors to go on strike, and if so, under what conditions?

This is another case where understanding some of the basic legal frameworks related to healthcare and medicine, in general, is useful, even before you evaluate the moral aspects of the question. Remember, there is no right or wrong answer; what's important is that you explain your thought process as you take into account the pillars of medicine. As you search your own ethical core for questions like this, always weigh the short- and long-term side effects and impact of what is being asked. If doctors strike, even for a single day, will anyone be harmed? Will someone go untreated? On the other hand, are there any structural issues that prevent providers from effectively treating patients? What responsibility do physicians have in advocating for change in their communities?

24. If the federal government asked you to suggest one positive change to immediately improve the healthcare system, what would you suggest?

Here's another question that speaks to your understanding and thoughtfulness as it relates to the broader healthcare system. Your answer here also displays your enthusiasm and optimism for working in a system that could be improved. Your ability to concisely articulate a positive change to this current system is the focus of this question.

It's also possible for a question like this to be posed to you in a role-playing scenario where you respond to a request from a government official who also debates the efficacy of your suggestion and discusses the merits and benefits of your idea. If that is the case, this is also an opportunity to demonstrate positively how you react and respond to constructive feedback.

25. Should doctors have a role in regulating full-contact sports like boxing, mixed martial arts, and professional football?

Here is another crossroads challenge that combines

medical ethics, current events, and legislation as it relates to professional sports. Should doctors, or other medical professionals, bring their knowledge, expertise, and informed opinions to the debate about safety regulations for full-contact sports? With a question like this, be sure to explore all options that would likely be available while also explaining the rationale behind your stance. It's also possible to have a range of answers conditional on the sport or factors at play (i.e., based on ages, duration of the activity, available safety equipment, and more...).

26. How do you feel about stem cell research using fetal tissue?

Health care is filled with moral, legal, and ethical issues that medical professionals face every day. Expect to have to answer tough questions like this that challenge the healthcare profession: abortion, assisted suicide, and cloning are a few of the other possible examples that an evaluator can reference. Speaking about this issue while considering medical ethics will demonstrate your critical thinking on the topic as well as your ability to discuss a complex and controversial issue in your own words. Remember that you don't need to understand the full science and technical aspects of each topic; your evaluator is assessing your ability to address the medical ethics components of the topic at your current level.

27. If you were granted a superpower, what would you want and why? (If you could GIFT this superpower to another person, who would you give it to and why?)

While this might seem like another light and fun question, you should realize that it reveals a lot about your worldview, maturity, passions, and aspirations. If given the same question but with the added stipulation of giving skill to another individual, you are being asked to be both

MOON PREP'S GUIDE TO MMI

thoughtful and altruistic while also demonstrating some logic behind your choice. As is the case with all other MMI questions, you should be adequately prepared to explain your line of reasoning behind your answer in either of the given scenarios.

28. Tell me your favorite quote and why you find it so meaningful.

This simple question is a way to reveal a guiding principle in your life; endorse the thoughts, teachings, or writings of a mentor; or reveal your ethical core through a quote that inspires you. It can be something simple, funny, enlightening, or inspiring, but you need to be able to clearly describe why it's your favorite and what impact it has on you.

29. Imagine a scenario in that, as a surgeon, you find out that your next patient is a convicted felon who has spent time in prison for a violent crime (for example assault and battery, murder, rape, child abuse, domestic abuse, etc.). What would you do?

In this situation, your exact actions and line of thinking are what the evaluators want to hear. Of course, you're being asked to respond to a scenario where you'd probably rather not know these details about your patient, but once you're aware of them, show just how you'd process them with your ethical and moral core. If this question is presented as a role-playing scenario, be prepared to share your plan of action while prioritizing your professionalism as a physician.

30. If you could immediately learn a skill that would typically take 5,000 or 10,000 hours to gain, what would you choose?

As you know, there are no shortcuts to skill acquisition, so this hypothetical question is more about what skills you most admire and why.. Like many others, your

43

answer here reveals complex things about your character, aspirations, work ethic, challenges, and plans.

It's also a question that speaks to self-awareness because you might decide that some skills would be better to build through the 10,000-hour learning process rather than any immediate boost. Whatever your choice may be in answering this question, be aware of its implications, and be prepared to adequately explain and support your response if needed.

31. Think about a mistake you've made that adversely impacted another person. Is it something you regret? What did you do in that situation that you might do differently now?

For many, speaking intelligently and candidly about past mistakes is very hard, especially if it's something you truly regret. It's an additional emotional challenge to discuss these mistakes if and when they harm others. Asking a medical school candidate to reflect on a poor choice from a past moment of their life and how their approach might be different now reveals much about their growth, maturity, and self-awareness.

In answering this question, it's important to remain composed while recounting the situation. You should be specific about your mistakes, but be sure to only include relevant details so that your evaluator can easily follow along with the story. Finish your answer on a positive note by highlighting what you have learned and how you have grown.

32. Are there any situations when it is okay for a physician to lie to a patient (Follow-up question: Have you told a white lie?)

This type of MMI question can be challenging because you have to dig deep and explore various avenues. It's okay if you conclude that there might be a situation where you think it is ethical to lie to a patient, but make sure to fully explain your thought process and the situation using the pillars of medicine to back up your response.

33. Do you think the priority of medicine should be about preventing disease by changing behavior or treating existing disease?

For these types of questions, you could respond either way; the most important aspect that you will be evaluated on is your ability to show your critical thinking skills and knowledge of healthcare. You may need to draw on your previous shadowing or volunteering experiences to formulate a well-rounded response. Be sure to also consider the current healthcare climate and what you have read when researching current healthcare issues.

34. Your colleague shows you a "Rate My Doc" site that allows patients to anonymously talk about their medical experience at your practice. Many of your patients have complained about your poor bedside manner and the unaffordability of your services. How would you react? (Follow up: Describe a time you received negative feedback. How did you respond?)

Here is another emotionally charged question that can either be asked directly or in a role-playing scenario. This type of difficult station is about your ability to display your personal growth when encountering tough feedback. People often get defensive when they feel like they might have done something wrong, so this is a window for the evaluator to get a sense of your core values, maturity, ethical and moral code, and experiences, even as a young person.

As in many of these types of emotionally charged questions, the intent might be to not only rattle you to the point of being fully candid but also to see how well you compartmentalize the experience as you move on to your next challenge. Be sure to take the time you need to process the question and gather your thoughts before starting your answer to avoid giving a flustered response.

For the follow-up questions, reflect on a past experience, sharing details about the situation but focusing mainly on the feedback and your subsequent response. Be sure to highlight how you have grown in that particular area since then.

5

SAMPLE MMI QUESTIONS FOR MEDICAL SCHOOL STUDENTS, PART TWO

The following prompts will involve more advanced knowledge of patient care. BS/MD students are not expected to have this type of advanced knowledge, and therefore, it is extremely unlikely they will encounter these types of questions during their interviews.

35. What is your take on the concept of Universal Basic Income (UBI)? (Follow up: Do you believe it would help or harm societies in general?)

A question like this assumes you know about the concept of UBI and have given some thought to how an income safety net program like this would play out in our society.

These general society and policy questions are a way to challenge your overall awareness of social issues that will come into play no matter where you practice medicine. It's also about having an opinion on a topic that may not be widely talked about. Expect that whether you support the initiative or not, it's likely that your evaluator

KRISTEN MOON

will take the other side of the "argument" to see how articulately and calmly you can handle stress, conflict, and differing opinions.

36. Describe your ideal career balance between clinical and research activities. (Follow up: Do you have any specific role models with this balance who you aspire to emulate?)

This is a tricky question that shows your understanding of how innovations, advancements, and breakthroughs are made in medicine and also how you imagine you'll be part of that. Can you clearly explain how you would ideally plan a career with hands-on clinical work and activity that was considered research? While there are pure researchers in medicine, it's almost a given that clinical medical professionals must continue their studies to remain current in their own field and specialty. Whether you would like to participate in that research itself is the core of the question.

The idea of role models here is tricky for some because before many candidates enter medical school, they may have no other medical role models other than their family's primary care physician. This is where extensive reading or shadowing physicians in your chosen field can fill the gap. Observing others or reading biographies of doctors, medical researchers, scientists, and others will give you a sense of what a life like this — balanced between clinical and research time—could look like.

37. A teenager [specifically a minor under age 17] asks you for a prescription for medical marijuana and also asks that you not mention the request to their parents or legal guardian. What would you do?

Here is another legal and ethical framework question where your best bet is to outline each response you'd make to this request and each individual step you'd take as you discuss the issue with your underage patient. What role does autonomy play here?

You'd also have to decide what aspects of this request you'd discuss with the parents or legal guardians and why. If questions like this seem difficult, then you've identified another area for further study and research before your MMI.

38. Imagine that it was your responsibility to rebalance an education budget in your state, and you must make emergency financial cuts. What would you remove and why?

Here is another broad policy question. While it is not about the healthcare system, it gives you a chance to display big-picture thinking skills, empathy, compassion, ethics, morality, as well as your critical thinking and communication skills. This is another question where you could expect that an evaluator could disagree with you on your choices just to see how you debate them and/or respond to the conflict.

39. You must choose between giving a liver transplant to a successful 60-year-old woman who actively volunteers in her community and a 24-year-old alcoholic. Who would you choose and why?

This ethical dilemma requires you to remain non-judgmental as you explain your thought process. You don't have to judge this prompt just on the small bit of information you see in the prompt. There are many more things you should be considering as you answer this type of prompt, including why the patients need the liver transplants, which patient is more likely to recover, and if the patients are even matches for the organ transplant.

When answering this question, you might want to rely on any guidelines the hospital might have in place already to address these types of issues. If there are

KRISTEN MOON

none, make sure to showcase ultimately what your response would be to make sure you remain fair in this decision.

40. A 25-year-old female comes into the ER with a nosebleed. You stop the bleeding, but she is now in a coma from blood loss and needs a transfusion to survive. However, the nurse finds a recent card from Jehovah's Witnesses Church stating that the patient refuses blood transfusions, regardless of the circumstances. What should you do?

Religious and cultural competency are key skills that a physician must display. Even if you don't agree with the patient and what they decide, you must rely on the ethical pillars of medicine to help you make a choice. Does the patient still have autonomy in this case? If, while shadowing, you had previous experiences while shadowing or volunteering with this type of situation, it is okay to use that story to back up your actions.

In your response, remember to remain respectful and understanding of a patient's wishes, regardless of what they are.

41. A company was hired by the government to develop a cure for the Ebola virus. They managed to successfully create a cure that reduces symptoms and the mortality rate for infected patients. What are the implications of this cure on a global scale?

Here's another question that speaks to your understanding of the healthcare system, not just in the U.S., but worldwide. Your ability to concisely articulate the various ramifications to patients around the world is being tested.

Make sure to look at the full picture: what are the ramifications of this vaccine for the patients who are affected? How will the vaccine be distributed? What roles would countries like the U.S. have in the distribution of this vaccine, especially to third-world countries?

Considering a wide perspective can help you answer this question more effectively.

42. A 25-year-old female patient with Down Syndrome is pregnant. Her husband and mother want her to get an abortion, but she does not. What should you do?

This question might seem more difficult when you first read it, but it requires similar skills that you've been practicing this whole time. The most important thing for you to consider is the competency level of the patient because she has Down Syndrome. One important thing to note about competency questions is to determine if the patient is legally dependent; if they are, they are deemed medically competent, and vice versa. Explain all sides of the issue and your thought process to display your soft skills to the elevators.

43. Explain the difference between Medicare and Medicaid.

This broad question is designed to make sure you have an understanding of the healthcare system and the difference between the two healthcare programs.

Pro tip: Medicare is "care" for the old while Medicaid is "aid" for the poor.

44. You are a genetic counselor. One of your clients, Meredith, had a baby girl with a genetic defect. All future pregnancies of Meredith have a chance of being affected by the same defect. You offered genetic testing on Meredith, her husband, and their daughter to find out more about their disease, to which everyone agreed. The result showed that neither Meredith nor her husband carries the mutation, but the girl inherited the mutation on a paternal chromosome that did not come from Meredith's husband. This means that the child's father might be unaware that he is a carrier of this disease. You suspect that both Meredith and her husband are aware of this non-paternity. How would you disclose the results of this genetic analysis to Meredith and her family?

What principles and who do you have to take into consideration in this case?

Longer prompts like this might seem overwhelming at first, but first, break down what you know and what is actually important for you to properly answer the prompt. Consider what your role as the physician is here —what should you say or do next?

These ethical dilemmas require you to consider the full picture and the repercussions of your actions. While confidentiality is not technically an ethical principle, it is loosely connected to several of them. Link whatever ethical principle drives you to your response to show-case your level of compassion and critical thinking skills.

45. A couple has decided to have a child through artificial insemination. They asked for the sex election of the child. What should a doctor advise in this situation?

This type of MMI prompt requires you to have some outside knowledge beforehand. As you prepare for the MMI, you should do your research on hot-button issues like artificial insemination to gain a better understanding of the issue.

As a physician, you shouldn't let your own personal beliefs sway the advice you give your patients but instead be driven by medical ethical principles. This station will test your ability to communicate clearly about difficult issues and take a definitive stance.

46. Dr. Young recommends homeopathic medicines and treat-ments to her patients. Despite the fact that there is no scientific evidence to show that homeopathic treatments work, Dr. Young continues to recommend the treatments to people with minor or non-specific symptoms such as muscle aches, headaches, or fatigue, even though she doesn't believe it is effective either. She does so because she believes there is no harm, and it reassures the patients.

What ethical problems does Dr. Young's behavior pose?

As you begin to formulate your response to your question, think about the ethical ramifications of these small white lies. While it might not be harming the patient, you should begin to consider what your ethical compass is.

In this situation, make sure to explain your exact thought process. Because this could be seen as an ethical gray area, you want to make sure that you are definitively choosing a side in your argument.

47. You are a family physician in a practice with four colleagues. Today is your day off, but at 4 PM, you receive a call from the nurse of a patient that lives in a nursing home and isn't doing well. His family had previously signed a do-not-resuscitate (DNR) order, but they are now reconsidering and want you to come immediately to discuss the situation and their options. However, you have already made a commitment to your family to attend an event together. What would you do?

This is not a trick question to see if you are a reliable worker or not; instead, this question wants you to deal with a tricky situation that doctors and healthcare patients face far too often. Not as a physician but as a human, you will need to clearly express what your priorities are at the moment.

As with many MMI dilemma questions, there is no one right answer. Someone's priorities might be different than yours, but as long as you talk through your thought process and try to find the best solution for all parties involved, then you will have answered the prompt correctly.

KRISTEN MOON

48. Due to the shortage of physicians in rural communities such as those in western states like North Dakota or Nebraska, some medical programs might prefer to admit students willing to work for two or three years in an underserved area once they graduate. What are the implications of this policy? Do you think this is effective?

This MMI question requires you to have an understanding of the healthcare landscape and awareness of issues surrounding the shortage of rural physicians. You are expected as a medical student to have basic knowledge of the healthcare system as a whole.

You may discuss the pros and cons of such a policy, including whether or not you think it is the duty of medical schools to serve their surrounding populations. Think of implications for medical students working in rural settings, such as lower pay to counteract student debt, along with benefits like lower burnout or access to a closer-knit community. This could be a good question to highlight your larger understanding of the role of physicians in society as public servants as well as individual doctors.

49. A 13-year-old girl is diagnosed with terminal brain cancer. She asks the doctors what her chances of survival are; however, her parents have asked the doctors not to tell her. What should the doctors do?

This is a tricky question, designed to get you to think about the rules around pediatric patients versus adult patients as well as considering patient autonomy. You are not obligated to disclose information to a minor if their parents disagree, but is that what is best for the patient? The answer is not so simple. Different cultures have different ideas about individual and family autonomy, which is important to recognize. Think out loud about

54

reasons why the parents would want to withhold information from their child; it usually has something to do with protective instinct, not maliciousness.

However, physicians are supposed to be advocates for their patients first and foremost, so while you may not go against the parents' wishes, you do have an obligation to have a conversation with the parents about their point of view, share the evidence around truth-telling, and compromise when indicated. But physicians are never required to lie, so consider asking the parents how they would want you to handle the patient's question. You can always defer any patient questions to them if you want to draw that line. "That's a really good question. Can we bring your parents in and have a conversation about it?"

On the flip side, if this were an adult patient, unless they explicitly tell you that they don't wish to know their prognosis, the family cannot dictate what they are told. Use this question to show your thought process and weigh the pros and cons openly to show conscientiousness.

50. You learn that one of your co-workers, who is also a physician, became sexually involved with a current patient who initiated or consented to the contact. What would you do? Is it ethical for a physician to become sexually involved with a patient?

This is one of the few questions that are not a gray area. Sexual involvement with a patient is a direct violation of the physician-patient relationship. If they want to continue to be involved, the physician-patient relationship must be dissolved first. However, while it can seem as simple as the patient getting a new physician, you may want to discuss the ethics of a possible informal lingering power dynamic within the relationship, which would display your thoughtfulness.

55

KRISTEN MOON

51. A 30-year-old schizophrenic patient needs surgery to repair a brain aneurysm. The surgeon discussed the procedure with the patient, who understood the procedure. Can the patient give consent?

Capacity is the ability of a patient to make medical decisions for themselves. Mental or cognitive issues do not automatically prevent patients from having capacity. Instead, it is a judgment made by the physician and is dictated by if the patient can understand the risks, benefits, and alternatives of any given decision/procedure. Capacity can change, even hourly, if a patient is acutely ill or delirious. While this patient has a mental illness and a brain issue, the question stem clearly states that they understood the procedure, so they can consent. You could even discuss the importance of avoiding stigmatizing mental health or cognitive disabilities within medicine, which would exhibit your compassion and maturity.

52. A 19-year-old female student is diagnosed to have suspected bacterial meningitis. She refuses further treatment and returns to the college dormitory. As the physician, what should you do?

This question wants you to think about autonomy and beneficence ("do good"). Competent patients have the right to refuse treatment or procedures, even if their life is in danger - autonomy trumps beneficence. However, physicians are obligated to inquire about reasons for non-compliance and attempt to alleviate them, educate and evaluate the patient for any suicidality or significant mental health concerns. You can discuss out loud the pros and cons of trying to treat this student outpatient, though oral antibiotics are extremely unlikely to be effective. Some physicians believe that something is better than nothing, while others want to prevent false reassurance

56

and protect their licenses. You can highlight the need for communication and persuasion skills as a physician and demonstrate empathy.

53. An 86-year-old terminally ill man calls to let you know he will be committing suicide by taking a lethal dose of painkillers. Before doing so, he wanted to let you know he appreciated all your help and let you know you had been a great doctor. How should you react in this situation?

While this is a difficult question to answer, you must pay careful attention to the facts here. For example, this does not fall under the category of physician-assisted suicide, and thus, no intervention or granting permission to the patient would not be acceptable. Further, in cases where someone is a potential danger to themselves or others, it is the physician's obligation to intervene. With this, you can also highlight your compassion, noting how you would comfort the patient while also ensuring they receive prompt medical care. Context is important here!

54. Suppose you are against abortion. A 17-year-old girl enters your office and acts for an abortion. What should you do?

Abortion is a tricky ethical issue, especially for providers. Knowing that you have a right to reject any patient for an abortion based on your beliefs is important in this scenario. Being rude or refusing to help further, however, is not acceptable. For this patient, remembering to refer her to another provider who will perform the procedure is important. Keep in mind: for anything related to sexual relations, drug/substance use, and mental health/relationships ("sex, drugs, and rock and roll" is a common saying used to remember this), you don't have to inform their parents if the patient is under 18-years-old. Expressing empathy and compassion in this setting despite your beliefs will also go a long way.

KRISTEN MOON

55. You have a 16-year-old patient with cancer. You've recommended chemotherapy, but the mom refuses treatment because she fears the chemotherapy won't help and it will make him sicker. What should you do?

Refusing treatment for a minor is a difficult situation to navigate for any provider, but there are specific steps that can be taken to ensure it is handled correctly. First, asking the parent what they know about the child's diagnosis and treatment options can be beneficial in (1) determining their baseline knowledge of the condition and (2) providing a platform for you to educate them. Explaining the diagnosis and benefits of chemotherapy in a compassionate, non-judgmental way can potentially help to convince them that the medication will significantly help their child.

However, if they still say no, you should remember that parents must act in the best interest of their children. This doesn't mean literally selecting the best drug or medication, but they must choose what they believe is the best option. Keep in mind in this scenario that context matters: parents may not refuse cancer treatment when withholding it causes harm to the patient and the benefits of it outweigh the risks or side effects. Acknowledging all of these factors in your discussion will impress your interviewer and ensure that you're fully answering the question.

56. You work in a clinic and one day, a patient comes in with her young child who has strep throat. As you are about to examine the child, the administrator calls you over and lets you know they are illegal immigrants with no insurance. Your clinic has already reached its quota of Medicare and Medicaid patients for the month. What should you do?

While the ethics and financial/logistic considerations

of the medical profession often come into conflict, it is important to understand all of the facts. First, physicians are required to provide care if it can endanger an individual's life, especially in children. Moreover, even if this isn't life-threatening, physicians are required to provide the necessary treatment for a given condition. While additional items (e.g., additional medications beyond the standard of care) aren't required, providing at least the minimum treatment for this patient is necessary. You can also go above and beyond the scope of the question and discuss aiding these individuals in finding organizations that can help them pay their medical bills.

Pro tip: when money and the care of a patient come into conflict, always put the patient first!

57. A patient is suing another doctor for medical malpractice. The patient, who has pancreatic cancer, comes to get treated by you; how would you react? Would you still see the patient?

This is a difficult question to answer for many physicians, let alone in an MMI. In general, (see #56), refusing to treat patients for financial reasons or a fear of being sued generally isn't the best course of action. Further, you cannot refuse treatment if denying a patient medications and/or procedures will cause harm to them. Additionally, speaking negatively about another doctor or discussing their mistakes is generally not advised, and thus, you should stay quiet about the lawsuit, even if the patient asks you about it. Discussing these factors can make you a standout interviewee on this question and demonstrate your knowledge of medical ethics.

58. How would you go about making the decision on whether or not to discontinue life support for a brain-dead patient?

Terminating life support for patients is never easy and is a sensitive subject for all providers. However, this deci-

KRISTEN MOON

sion is not the physician's to make - it depends on the patient's code status as well as those closest to the patient. If a patient is not "Do Not Resuscitate (DNR)" or "Do Not Intubate (DNI)," you must go to the patient's next of kin. However, instead of placing the decision immediately on the family or healthcare proxy, it is critical that they understand the full prognosis of their loved one. Many families do not understand or fully deny that their loved one will not return to a healthy state. Therefore, educating them and ensuring they understand this fact will provide for more open communication. Moreover, involving palliative care in this discussion can provide an extra layer of understanding and compassion during this difficult decision. Should the family still refuse to end life support after these meetings, you must accept their decision. However, checking in regularly with them without being pushy is acceptable and the best course of action. General tip: Do not impose your beliefs onto patients or their families.

Next up, let's talk about being fully prepared for your interviews.

6

BE FULLY PREPARED FOR
THE MMI

Now that you've seen a range of sample questions, you have a sense of what the MMI challenges can be. Your experience with MMI may cover none of these topics or some variation of them. So, to be fully prepared for the interviews, expect a full range of challenges, in various formats, related to these common topics for MMI scenarios:

Vaccines, abortion, terminal illness, cultural competency, cheating, stealing, teamwork, why medicine, explaining the differences between Medicare and Medicaid, current topics/issues in the healthcare system, end of life care, safe injection programs, personal challenge questions (why this med school, personal experiences, etc.); and wildcard questions (for example, having to sit back to back with someone and do origami.)

Essentially, if you can imagine a question, scenario, or challenge in the context of these medical school interviews, be prepared for it.

61

- Standard interviews: the traditional sit-down interview with one or more medical school admissions professionals, a department head, or another recruiting staff member.
- Ethical scenarios with complex social and/or policy implications. These are often connected to current events, legal frameworks in your jurisdiction, specific policy issues (current or proposed), and public health topics and concerns. Having a foundational basis to discuss these types of subjects clearly and succinctly is extremely useful.
- Interactions with a role-playing actor portraying a patient, an authority figure, a family member, or a loved one (this will likely only occur with in-person interviews).
- Rest station for taking a break. Don't underestimate the importance of this part of your MMI schedule. Strategically, this is also a moment for an emotional reset of all your interactions in prior scenarios.

As you've seen in the sample questions, they often give applicants challenging questions meant to rattle their reactions and responses just to see how they handle conflict, stressful situations, adversity, opposing opinions, and more. Even the recovery time after a conflict is something often observed by evaluators.

If an applicant—rattled by a prior scenario—is finding it difficult to focus on a new task at hand, this person is revealing that they might not have the ability to compartmentalize the difficulties, stress, and emotional toll of being a physician. The interviewers are often trained to push back on your answers too. You have to be prepared for them to argue with you and defend your position. Essentially, they want to see if you'll waiver in the face of criticism or questioning. Just knowing that the ability to let go of previous stations (i.e., any difficulties, conflicts, and your responses) is a useful strategy that has helped many applicants.

But remember this. It's what keeps far too many applicants from preparing fully for their MMI. The most damaging rumor about the medical school applicant's (MMI) interview process is clearly that there are no wrong answers. You know that it's not true. And those who believe that there are no wrong answers and can say whatever comes to mind at the moment are the candidates who often don't prepare for their MMI process. And then regret it.

You can even prepare in the moments prior to entering the MMI room as well. Most programs will provide you with a pen and paper meant to organize your thoughts. Taking an extra 30 seconds can actually go a long way in terms of helping you plan and organize your answer. Many applicants fall into the trap of "word vomiting" in order to fill the time in a given room. That is the wrong strategy. Mapping out 3-5 examples or supporting details that provide evidence for your position will impress your interviewer with both your knowledge and ability to organize your thoughts coherently.

Clearly, there are wrong answers. Especially if you face a scenario that presents a moral or ethical dilemma, and your answers don't show honesty, integrity, professionalism, or authentic care and empathy for patients, they will not offer you a slot in their medical school program. Even a brilliant response poorly communicated would result in a less-than-stellar evaluation.

Time is your biggest ally as a medical school student. Use your time wisely. You now have a workable MMI prep strategy as you enter the critical evaluation process of medical school admissions. May the work, study, and self-discovery you do before your first evaluation open doors for you to make your dreams of a career in medicine move one step closer. Good luck in medical school!

7

LIST OF MEDICAL SCHOOLS USING MMI IN THEIR ADMISSIONS PROCESS

To assist you in your career planning, here is a partial list of United States, Puerto Rican, and Canadian medical schools which require the MMI as part of their current application process. Be sure to confirm the most up-to-date admissions process at any institution where you plan to apply to understand their latest requirements for your medical school, BS/MD, and BS/DO application. Please visit our site moonprep.com for other helpful resources.

- Albany Medical College
- California Northstate University College of Medicine
- Central Michigan University College of Medicine
- Chicago Medical School at Rosalind Franklin University of Medicine & Science
- Dalhousie University Faculty of Medicine

- Donald and Barbara Zucker School of Medicine at Hofstra/Northwell
- Duke University School of Medicine
- Faculty of Medicine Université Laval
- Kaiser Permanente School of Medicine
- Max Rady College of Medicine at the University of Manitoba
- McGill University Faculty of Medicine
- McMaster University Michael G. DeGroote School of Medicine
- Medical College of Georgia at Augusta University
- Memorial University of Newfoundland Faculty of Medicine
- Michigan State University College of Human Medicine
- New York Medical College
- New York University Long Island School of Medicine
- New York University School of Medicine
- Northern Ontario School of Medicine
- Nova Southeastern University Dr. Kiran C. Patel College of Allopathic Medicine
- Oregon Health & Science University School of Medicine
- Queen's University School of Medicine
- Rutgers Robert Wood Johnson Medical School
- San Juan Bautista School of Medicine
- Stanford University School of Medicine
- SUNY Upstate Medical University College of Medicine
- TCU and UNTHSC School of Medicine

- University of Toledo College of Medicine and Life Sciences
- Universidad Central del Caribe School of Medicine
- Universite de Montreal Faculty of Medicine
- Universite de Sherbrooke Faculty of Medicine
- University of Alabama School of Medicine
- University of Alberta Faculty of Medicine and Dentistry
- University of Arizona College of Medicine – Tucson
- University of Arizona College of Medicine – Phoenix
- University of British Columbia Faculty of Medicine
- University of Calgary Cumming School of Medicine
- University of California, Davis School of Medicine
- University of California, Los Angeles David Geffen School of Medicine
- University of California, Riverside School of Medicine
- University of California, San Diego School of Medicine
- University of Cincinnati College of Medicine
- University of Illinois College of Medicine
- University of Massachusetts Medical School
- University of Minnesota Medical School
- University of Mississippi School of Medicine
- University of Missouri – Kansas City School of Medicine

- University of Nevada Reno School of Medicine
- University of Saskatchewan College of Medicine
- University of South Carolina School of Medicine – Greenville
- University of Texas at Austin Dell Medical School
- University of Utah School of Medicine
- University of Vermont Larner College of Medicine
- Virginia Commonwealth University School of Medicine
- Virginia Tech Carilion School of Medicine
- Wake Forest School of Medicine
- Washington State University Elson S. Floyd College of Medicine
- Wayne State University School of Medicine
- Western Michigan University Homer Stryker M.D. School of Medicine

ABOUT THE AUTHOR

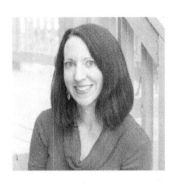

Kristen Moon is a leading national authority on medical school admissions for Direct Medical Programs and traditional MD and DO. As the founder and CEO of Moon Prep, an educational consultancy, Kristen leads a team of dedicated and trusted professionals that deliver on a clear mission: partnering with ambitious students to prepare them for a successful journey into medicine. With a particular focus on MD, BS/MD, and BS/DO programs, Kristen has assembled a team of experienced independent counselors and mentors who build long-term relationships with students and their families, carefully advising them one-on-one through the entire application process.

What started as working with only a handful of students each year, has since grown to dozens of counselors distributed across the United States, working with hundreds of aspiring medical students across the world. The Moon Prep teams partner with these aspiring medical students to navigate the challenging admission requirements and focus on crafting compelling applications that convince, inspire, and leave a lasting impression on the admission committees of their top-choice programs. As the author of *BS/MD Programs: A Comprehensive Guide* and a regular contributor to *Forbes*, Kristen's highly-sought expertise has also been featured in leading outlets such as the *U.S. News & World Report, Investopedia, Mass Mutual, Apple News, Inc.*, and more.

Kristen resides in Atlanta, Georgia with her husband, Rok, and their daughters Zoe and Sophie. She holds an MBA from Emory University's Goizueta Business School and a BS in Engineering from Stony Brook University. In her spare time, you'll find her biking on the Silver Comet Trail and hiking Kennesaw Mountain.

www.moonprep.com

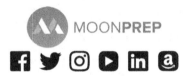

ALSO BY KRISTEN MOON

BS/MD Programs: A Comprehensive Guide

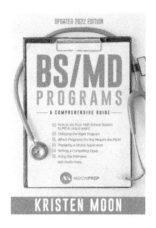

Made in the USA
Las Vegas, NV
21 December 2023

83431284R00052